GW00498979

Good Housekeeping

make
the
most of
your eyes

Jo Glanville-Blackburn

series editor
Vicci Bentley

HarperCollins*Illustrated*

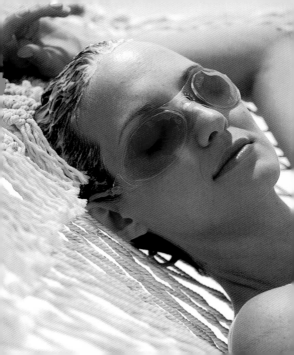

contents

introducing eyes [6]

looking after eyes [14]

making-up eyes [44]

the final frame [88]

step-by-step eyes [104]

'discretion
is being able to
raise your
eyebrow instead
of your voice.'

Anon

4

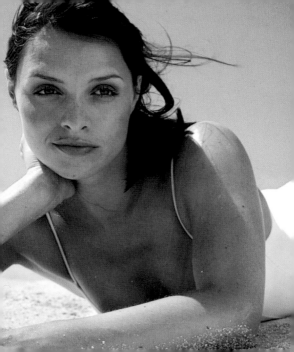

Your eyes can tell more about the way you feel than any other part of your body. Your eyes can express sadness and joy, passion or indifference, fatigue or a sudden zest for life, all within the blink of an eye and without even uttering a single word. Close them slightly and you are mistrusting, raise a single brow and you are a vamp, then crinkle them slightly to show that you were only joking.

6

introducing eyes

Eyes mirror what is in your heart and reflect the way you feel. The colour of the eye itself is said to give a good indication of your true personality. Some experts believe that dark-eyed people are generally business-minded, work well under great pressure and tend to use their initiative; while pale-eyed people have more stamina, but may be more sentimental and moody, and are inclined to be better at reading.

'stay clean and bright ... you are the window through which you must see the world.'

George Bernard Shaw

8

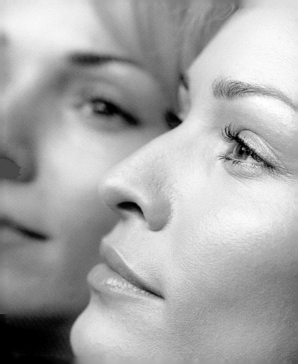

Look even deeper and iridolo-
gists (eye-health specialists)
claim to be able to diagnose a
variety of illnesses such as
arthritis and digestive prob-
lems just by examining the iris
10   (the coloured part of the eye).
Little wonder when you
consider how our general
health, diet and daily lifestyle
is reflected in our eyes. A lack
of quality sleep for just one or
two nights instantly takes its
toll, just as a brisk walk in the

fresh air will revitalise your body and soul and put a healthy glint and sparkle back into your eyes.

Make sure to drink the recommended eight glasses of water each day, and you can be sure to see the results in your eyes. Attitude counts for a lot too: laughter and positive thinking shows in your every expression and puts a light in your eye that those around you admire and adore.

'i am a dreamer
... one who can find
his way by
moonlight, and see
the dawn before the
rest of the world.'

Oscar Wilde

12

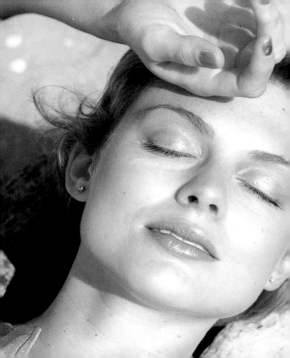

the skin around your eyes
is very sensitive and
vulnerable. It is the first
place to show wrinkles
and will need
extra daily care
and protection.

looking

after eyes

The skin around the eye is incredibly fine and delicate compared to the skin on the rest of the face. At 0.5 mm thick – a quarter the depth of most skin on the body – it more readily absorbs UV light, which damages the skin. The skin around the eye has less collagen and elastin to keep it supple and stretchy, and loses moisture more quickly than anywhere else on the body. Your eyes express your emo-

skin around the eyes

tional state as well as reacting to light, sun, wind, smoke and cold. A total of 22 muscles are constantly reacting to emotional and physical stimuli.

We often forget and rarely appreciate the extraordinarily clever mechanisms that operate and protect our eyes. The eyes are guarded by the eyelids which automatically close to protect the surface of the eye from injury and which keep a fresh supply of fluid across the cornea as we continuously blink. Tears help to wash away small irritants which land in the eye. Eyelashes too, a delicate extension of the eyelids, provide extra protection from dust and debris.

The rules for eye health are pretty basic. Eyes must be protected from strain, glare, dust and dirt. Just like the rest of the body they need relaxation at frequent intervals. Sun exposure accounts for 90 per

cent of wrinkles and so they
need extra protection from UV
light. Lack of sleep, exercise
and fresh air all result in dull,
tired eyes. As does a poorly
balanced diet. The right foods
are in the vitamin A group,
found in citrus fruits, apricots,
green leafy vegetables, carrots,
turnips, egg-yolks, butter and
cheese. For clear and sparkling
eyes, drink more water, avoid
too much alcohol and sun, and
do not smoke.

Do eat an antioxidant-rich diet with lots of fresh foods and oily fish.

Do regularly apply cream to the eye area. You don't need to use a specific eye product, but if you do you are less likely to get watery or puffy eyes which often result from cream slipping into the eyes.

20

Do get regular eye checks, annually if you already wear glasses or contact lenses. Get a check-up if your eyes feel itchy, burning or drier than usual.

the do's and don'ts

- Do work out where exactly you need to apply eye cream – find your laugh lines by scrunching-up your eyes – and apply cream over the whole area.

- Don't smoke. It's bad for your skin and your health, robs the body of essential nutrients, makes eyes tired and sore, and releases free-radicals throughout the body which are renowned for their ageing effects on the skin.

Don't drag or pull the delicate skin around the eye when you are cleansing and moisturising. Gently dab gels or creams on to the surrounding area.

Tip: if you smudge your mascara or eye-shadow, don't remove the whole make-up, just dip a cotton bud into a little eye make-up remover lotion and lightly dab away.

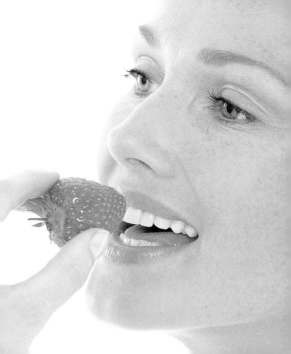

Removing eye make-up can be a bit like removing red wine from a white carpet. But better to remove make-up than to sleep in it, which is both unhygienic and bad for the eye itself. Your regular facial cleanser may irritate your eyes, so choose one specifically designed for the job, preferably oil-free, especially if you wear contact lenses.

The most effective way to remove mascara is to soak a

cleansing your eyes

cotton-wool ball in eye make-up remover lotion, hold against the lashes and lightly press into them to absorb the make-up. Then stroke downwards without tugging and pulling at the eyelid. Rubbing is especially hard on the eyes and surrounding skin, and makes it more likely that the cleanser will leak into your eye. If you plan to re-apply eye make-up immediately afterwards, an oil-free remover won't leave any

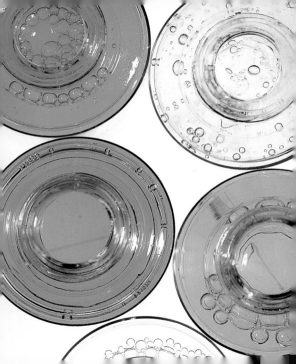

residue. Always remove contact lenses before removing eye
make-up, and don't handle
lenses unless your fingertips
are clean and dry.

For sore, tired eyes – soak and chill two chamomile tea bags (used ones are fine), lie down and place on closed lids for 10 minutes to soothe. (Ordinary tea bags will do fine too.)

To wake up sleepy eyes – place two cotton-wool balls, which have been soaked in ice cold milk, over your eyes for five minutes.

To soothe red, sore, itchy eyes – add a few drops of 'Eyebright' into a glass of water and drink throughout the day. It is the best herbal remedy for eyes.

trouble-shooting eyes

- To take the heat out of skin and to reduce puffiness – beauty therapist, Janet Filderman, suggests wrapping a small ice-cube in a handkerchief and gliding it over the face from the inside corner of the nose to the ear and down the side to just under the jaw. Repeat on both sides.

- To reduce dark circles often caused by stress, fatigue and, in some cases, hereditary – make an effort to go to bed an hour earlier, drink more water and reduce your intake of dairy foods.

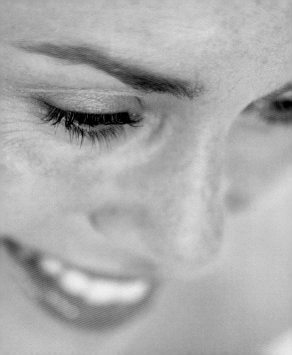

To reduce puffiness around the eyes –
try sleeping with an extra pillow and lie
on your back, to help prevent fluids
from 'pooling' around the eyes.

To reduce 'crow's feet' – make sure you
regularly apply eye gel or cream and
wear sunglasses. Even in winter the sun
can make you squint, especially when
driving, so invest in a good pair which
offer 100 per cent UV protection.

Soothing eye bath

25 g (1 oz) dried Eyebright leaves • 600 ml
(1 pint) hot water • cotton-wool pads
Steep the leaves in the hot water, allow to cool,
then dip two cotton-wool pads in the solution.
Wipe eyes if they need clearing of a foreign

object, then place two more soaked pads on
your eyes and relax for 10–15 minutes. You can
drink the tea too.

eye-pack recipes

Chilled eye compress

slices of chilled raw potato • muslin squares
Place slithers of raw potato between two pieces
of gauze and place over your eyes as a cooling
compress. You can use chilled cucumber too.

Brightening eye tonic

1 tbsp cool chamomile tea • 1 tbsp witch hazel
• ½ tsp castor oil • 1 drop frankincense oil
Mix the tea and witch hazel together in a clean
jar, then add the oils. Shake well to mix. Store in
the fridge and use whenever eyes are tired and
sore, by dipping cotton wool pads into the
solution and resting on the eyes for 10 minutes.

Moisturising balm

I tsp avocado oil • I tsp wheatgerm oil • I tsp calendula oil • ½ tsp honey • tiny blob of cocoa butter

Place the ingredients in a heat-proof bowl, and place the bowl in a saucepan of hot water. Heat until ingredients have melted together, transfer the mixture into a clean, airtight container and use in place of your night cream.

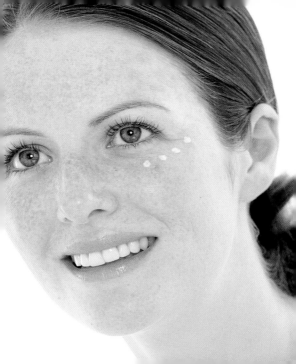

Make your eyes appear alive and beautiful even if you have had less than the recommended eight-hours sleep. Doing eye exercises helps to pull the fluid down from around the eye area so that unsightly puffiness and bags are eliminated swiftly. They work both by stimulating the skin's micro-circulation (a delicate network of veins and capillaries that boost freshly oxygenated blood through the skin), and also on specific acu-

exercises for tired eyes

pressure points around the eyes that hold tension and stress in everyday expressions. And while you might think that repeatedly scrunching your eyes up will only give you more wrinkles, the fact is that eye exercises are rated as a real boost, helping to improve muscle tone, eliminate puffiness and boost circulation. Plus these cost nothing to do, and you can easily do them anywhere you choose.

raise your upper lids and eyebrows opening your eyes as wide as possible, at a rate of one per second. Repeat 15 times. Look straight ahead, slowly raise your lower eyelids. Repeat 15 times. Close your eyes and look down behind the lids. Put your index finger on the centre of each upper lid, and try to open your eyes 10 times, keeping the lids closed with your fingertips.

38

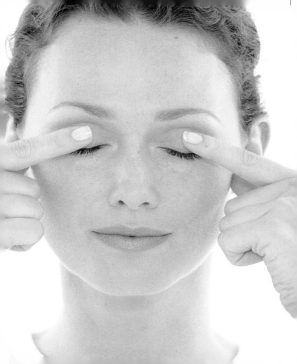

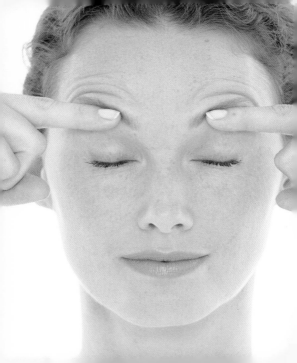

Exercise to lift droopy eyelids – look straight ahead and place each index finger lengthwise under your brows, then push them up using your fingers and hold them firmly against the bone. With your fingers still in place, close your eyelids very slowly, feeling the pull from brow to lashes. Still in this position, squeeze your eyes together and hold for a count of three, then open and relax. Repeat this exercise five times.

Relieve a headache – sit looking straight ahead. Open and close your eyes 10 times at a rate of one per second. Face straight ahead, look to your far left with your eyes only and slowly roll your eyes up and over to the far right. Roll them back again to the left. Repeat five times. Next, look to your far left, then slowly roll your eyes down and across to the far right. Roll back to the left and repeat five times.

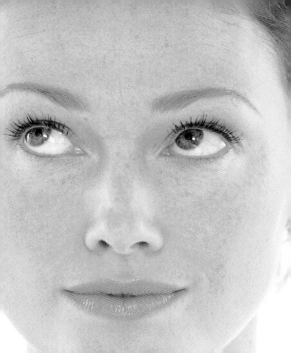

eye make-up
should be a soft haze
of colour, apply
subtle, natural
tones and you will
look fresh,
warm and appealing.

making

p eyes

Make-up brushes are often considered as just an accessory for when you have time to play around with make-up, but the truth is that with the right tools your make-up goes from passable to professional. Powders glide onto the skin and blend seamlessly, shading and contouring, rather than sitting in an obvious layer. Make-up artists agree on the following six basic eye essentials.

A shadow brush: a short brush, cut full and square for a clean sweep of colour.

basic eye kit

- A liner brush: a small flat brush which is gently rounded to a point.
- A brow brush: this brush has firm bristles, clipped into an angle, to allow the application of a clean, even powder of shadow on the brows.
- Metal slanted tweezers: these angled tweezers rarely miss a single hair.
- Eyelash curlers: to neaten lashes into line and curl them so they open up the eyes.
- A metal eyelash comb: to remove any clumps of mascara and separate lashes perfectly.

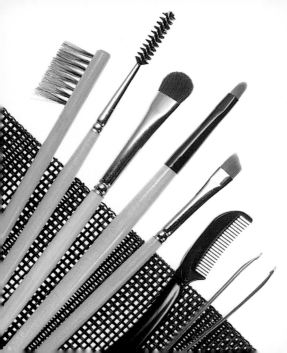

'having a good set of brushes is the key to professional looking eye make-up... '

Bobbi Brown, make-up artist

For longer-lasting, crease-proof eye-shadow, it is important to prime your skin properly with sheer translucent face powder before applying eye make-up. Avoid using eye cream immediately prior to making-up as it will cause the eye-shadow to crease within seconds, allow about 15 minutes for it to be fully absorbed first.

Smooth out your skin tone and cover any bluish veins with foundation, then, using a

priming your face

velour powder puff, pat the eyelids with face powder. Apply a matte eye-shadow that matches your skin tone and blend across the entire eyelid, from lashes to brow, using a shadow brush.

Now you can apply any shade of powder eye-shadow you choose. It will now blend beautifully in a wash of colour that you can build up for more intensity, in the confidence that it will stay in place longer.

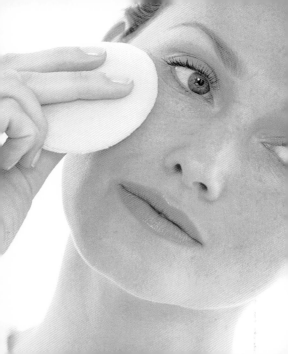

'prime the eyelids with an undercoat of foundation and powder ... shape and contour from this simple canvas.'

Maggie Hunt, make-up artist

The true art of make-up is in learning how to conceal the things you don't want to see, and highlighting the bits you do. Concealers are great at hiding blemishes, and many make-up artists favour using concealer alone so that skin is kept as fresh and natural as possible. Apply with a fine brush and you can literally paint out imperfections such as thread veins, ageing lines and even spots.

concealer and highlighte

When matching the right concealer to your skin, choose a
colour that is one shade lighter
than your foundation. If it's
too pale it will show up imperfections even more.

To conceal bags under the
eyes, put concealer on the
shadow beneath the bag, not
on it – or you will be highlighting rather than concealing the
bags. When you want to cover
dark circles, look ahead in a
mirror, put your chin down to

show the darkness up even more, then paint concealer onto the dark shadows only.

Highlighters are powders or creams for the face and eyes which contain shimmering microparticles of titanium dioxide to catch the light and enhance natural 'highs' such as the brow-bones, cheek-bones and lips. Because they highlight rather than conceal, they will highlight flaws in the skin if applied inappropriately.

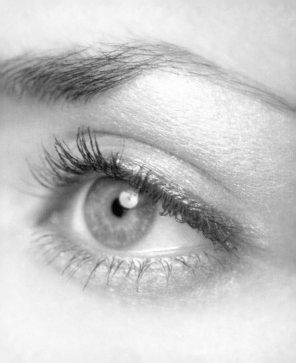

You can't change the shape of your eyes, but with eye-shadow you can create the illusion of bigger, wider, narrower or deeper eyes with just a little clever shading and contouring. It's one of the most useful items of make-up and one we rarely use to its full potential. So if you're feeling in the middle of a make-up rut, now is the time to experiment. Just changing your make-up will reawaken your face and take years off it.

eye-shadow

For the most modern look, keep your eye make-up simple. A clean sweep of a single colour, matte or shimmering, is just about all you need for a basic daytime look. Then experiment a little more for evening, using shadows to shape your eyes for more definition. Remember that mattes are best for contouring, while iridescent shadows work as highlighters. Use dark shadows to create depth and to make

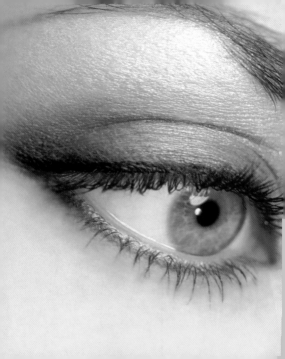

prominent areas recede, and light shadows to emphasise and make less prominent areas of the eye stand out.

Most make-up artists consider that almond-shaped eyes are the ideal shape to make-up. However, if your eyes are small or close-set, there are some useful tricks to try when applying shadow. Now turn the page to find out which colour eyeshadow suits your colouring.

There is only one reliable way to truly gauge what your best colours are: they must do something for you – bringing your eye or hair colour alight.

Blond hair

blue-grey eyes	taupe over lids
	brown to contour
brown eyes	green over lids
	deeper green to contour
green eyes	grey-blue over lids
	grey to contour

Red hair

blue-grey eyes	peach over lids
	mid-brown to contour
brown eyes	grey-green over lids
	heather to contour
green eyes	lilac over lids, blue to contour

shades for natural colou

Brown or black hair

blue-grey eyes	lilac over lids heather to contour
brown eyes	pale grey over lids slate-grey to contour
green eyes	pale lilac over lids blue-grey to contour

Grey hair

blue-grey eyes	taupe over lids heather to contour
brown eyes	lilac over lids heather to contour
green eyes	pale blue over lids grey to contour

63

If your eyes are close-set – concentrate light colours on the inner corners and darker shades on the outer edges of your eyes.

If your eyes are wide-set – do the opposite, concentrate dark shadows on the inner corners and light shadows on the outer corners.

To lift droopy lids – shade the outer corners of the eyes, tapering colour upwards and outwards.

trouble-shooting shadow

- To enhance small eyes – avoid dark shadows and concentrate shading colour on the socket lines and outer edges. White pencil along the inner lower lid will also make the whites of the eye look bigger and brighter.

- For longer lasting shadow – put powder eye-shadow on with a damp brush. The shadow will dry into the skin as you blend it, and because it clings to the wet brush you'll avoid the problem of dry eye-shadow crumbling onto your cheek.

To avoid eye-shadow falling on your skin – apply a heavy dusting of loose powder on your cheek. It will catch any falling debris and you can then brush it away leaving your make-up intact.

66

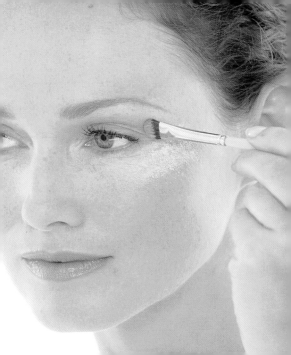

Eyeliner gives eyes **extra definition and becomes almost indispensable with age as lashes become sparse and eyes become deeper set. If you are looking for a more subtle, smoky looking eye that doesn't look harsh and obvious, choose a kohl eyeliner pencil. Pencils are especially good for those who are wary of eyeliner as you can build the line up gradually and blend it softly away if it starts to look heavy.**

eyeliner pencils

The best way to apply pencil liner is one third of the way along from the inner corner of the eye close to the lashes, tapering up and off at the corners. Then smudge-blend to get the degree of depth you want. For a really subtle eyeliner application, pull back the eyelid a little and fill in between the lashes from underneath. The effect is amazing. Instead of using an eyeliner sharpener, sharpen eye pencils

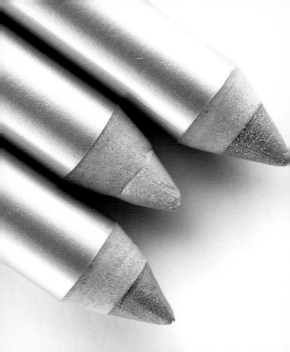

with a razor blade, shaving repeatedly from top to bottom on one side and then again on the opposite side. The result is a rectangular tip that allows for a much cleaner line between the lashes.

It takes practice to apply liquid eyeliner well, but the overall effect is much more dramatic than with a pencil. However, because it gives a very definite line, it can look a little harsh on older skin and tends to look more flattering on younger eyes which are smoother and less crêpey.

The trick to applying perfect eyeliner is to look down into a mirror lying flat on a table in front of you. This way you can

eyeliner liquids

see the whole eyelid, have both hands free, and you can rest your elbow on the table to steady your hand. Try a variety of shades. If you have blue eyes, brown or navy eyeliner looks softer and prettier than black. If you have brown eyes, then a dark brown or cocoa shade looks more subtle and if you have green eyes try brown or charcoal liner.

If eyeliner makes your eyes look smaller – add white kohl pencil on the inner rim of your eye. It's a theatrical trick that makes the white of the eye appear bigger. If you always get a wobbly line – keep your elbows steady on a table, looking down into a mirror and stretch the skin along the lid before applying, so you have a smooth surface. Don't give up – practice makes perfect.

trouble-shooting eyeline

If your liquid eyeliner smears or blobs –
dip a cotton bud in a little eye make-up
remover lotion and stroke away the
mark. Powder and blend again. Now you
should be able to finish where you first
left off.

If your pencil liner rubs off too quickly –
try painting liquid liner underneath
first. Then draw over the top with pencil
and smudge-blend to get the softness.
This also gives the pencil something to
cling to, making it last longer.

If the point of your eye pencil breaks off while you're sharpening it – it means that the pencil is too soft. So put it in the fridge for an hour or two before sharpening to make it harder and therefore less likely to break.

76

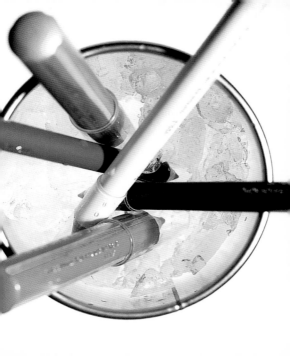

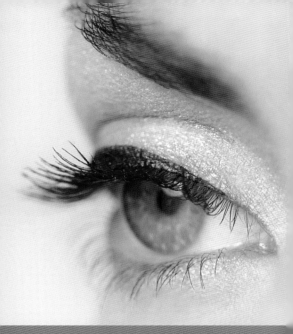

mascara

Mascara thickens and emphasises your lashes, in fact eyes look positively naked without it. You can even select your ideal mascara type, from lash-building mascaras, which contain filaments to thicken; to lash-lengthening which often contain polymers for a natural, glossy finish; to water-resistant, long-lasting formulas.

Mascara brushes come in a variety of styles too and can make a difference to the finished effect.

Graduated bristles suit longer lashes and give a 'spiky' look.

Curved bristles coat all the lashes at once, but often miss the roots.

Straight and slim bristles are great for hard to reach lashes.

Spiral bristles are good for short or fine lashes and don't overload the lashes.

Hollow-fibre bristles hold lots of colour so you get a thicker application for more volume.

mascara tools

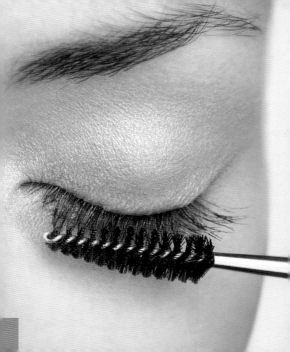

To apply your mascara, wipe the wand with a tissue first, if the first coat is too heavy, your eyelashes will stick together. Next, brush the upper lashes downwards from the top, and the lower lashes upwards from underneath. Apply sparingly: it is very easy to overdo it on the first coat and then your lashes will look caked, stuck together and totally false. Finish by brushing through any lumps with a mascara comb (preferably metal) to separate lashes.

Tip: if you want to use eye-lash curlers to make your lashes appear thicker and longer, curl before applying mascara or the tongs will cling to the mascara and pull the lashes. Look down, clamp the top lashes between the tongs and wait for approximately 30 seconds before releasing them.

To prevent clumpy lashes – wipe your mascara brush with a tissue before you use it, it's not a waste and if you wipe it on the side of the tube, it will clump even more quickly.

If your mascara always smudges – leave it off the bottom lashes. If it still smudges, it might not be a good formulation, so try a different make. Ask friends for their recommendations.

84

- If you have pale lashes and can't reach the lash base with your mascara wand – use liquid eyeliner in a matching shade to paint on the bits you've missed.
- If you've blobbed your mascara – use a clean damp mascara wand to separate clogged lashes and a damp cotton-bud to clean blobs from the skin.
- If you suffer from any eye infection, styes or conjunctivitis – don't throw your mascara away. Never lend your mascara to anyone either.

If your eyes smart after using your regular mascara – it's probably time to throw it out. Mascaras only tend to last around three months at the most.

Make sure you always curl your eyelashes before using mascara or your tongs will cling to your lashes.

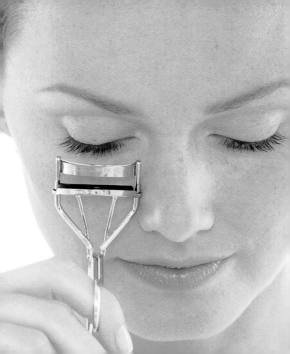

eyebrows influence
the balance, feel and
character of a face fa
more than any other
single
feature.

the fina

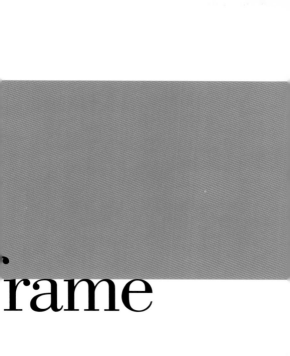

rame

Eyebrows are the most under-rated part of your face, yet with the right shaping they make a huge difference to your looks, making you look bright-eyed and years younger. The arch, shape and width of your eyebrows will determine the expression on your face – and to some extent your mood and the way people perceive your mood to be.

Neat brows enhance the shape of your eyes. If eyebrows are

your ideal shape

shaped to balance the rest of the face, your eyes will automatically appear bigger. To get the shape of your brows right, hold a pencil alongside your nose. The inner edge of your eyebrow should start vertically above the inner corner of your eye. Now lay the pencil from the outside edge of your nostril past the outer corner of your eye, where it touches is where the brow should end.

The arch of your brow should

be about half way along your eye socket, just beyond the outer edge of the iris. If you are still unsure check the shape before you begin by drawing over the hairs you want to pluck with a white pencil. Bear in mind that a new shape is high-maintenance and may need weekly or bi-weekly touch-ups. Use tweezers with an angled head and a fine tip to create a definite shape and for a general tidy-up.

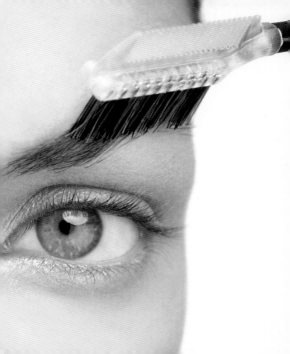

Eyebrows have, over the years, swung from pencil thin to thick and 'natural' and back again. The current trend of letting your natural eyebrow shape be your guide is the most flattering. Take your time and use a magnifying mirror in daylight. To shape brows properly, pluck one hair at a time from underneath the natural brow line. Never shape the top hairs or they will end up patchy and unbalanced. Pull each hair out

how to pluck eyebrows

with a swift, sharp tug in the direction it is growing, while holding the skin taut.

Comb brows into shape, take a good look at where you want to pluck. Tidy-up obvious stray hairs – this may be all you need to do. To make a more definite shape, keep using the pencil as your rule. As you pluck, step back and make sure each brow matches the other – do a few hairs on one side then some on the other so that they balance.

This is especially important if you have fair colouring as the colour of your eyebrows tends to fade as you get older. So, if your brows are pale, thin or sparse, fill in with a eyebrow pencil that matches the natural colour of your eyebrows or is a tone lighter. Eyebrow pencils are firmer than eye-shadow pencils so they are less likely to smudge.

Draw colour in with tiny, upward feathery strokes in the

correcting with colour

direction of hair growth, and subtly extend the line. Then blend with a stiff brow brush, working the colour through the brows upwards and outwards, following the shape of the natural brow-line.

If you've over-plucked and your brows are too thin, grow them back and use a mushroom coloured powder-shadow to enhance them. Decide which areas need filling in with pencil and resist the urge to pluck

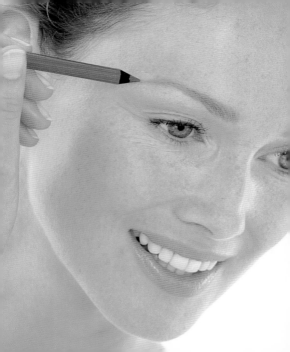

new hairs growing through. When using shadow, tap off your brush any excess powder so you don't overdo it. Apply colour to the arch first then go back to the inner edge and taper off to the end. This way you won't end up with a heavy looking brow which is hard to remedy afterwards.

If you have very pale brows, groom them so they follow the shape of your eyes. Blondes often have lots of light baby hairs. If you are unsure about where to start, try drawing the shape you want with a pencil and use it as a guide. Once shaped, they will look tidy and can be coloured in or dyed.

Keep the colour light to compliment your hair.

To help low eyebrows appear higher, brush eyebrows downwards so you can see exactly where the uppermost hairs emerge from the skin. With a pencil or eye-shadow and brush, trace along this upper limit, emphasising the highest part of your brow line, then when you brush the hairs up, you will have a neatly hidden pencil line.

If you find plucking too painful – do ice your brows before plucking to numb the pain or try a little baby teething gel which contains an anaesthetic. Tea tree oil will reduce any irritation. Plucking after a shower or bath is often less painful because the skin is softer.

If your eyebrows are untidy – do make sure they are well-groomed and try a clear eyebrow gel to keep hairs in place.

If your eyebrows look too heavy – do brush a clean mascara wand through them to diffuse the pencil tone.

do's and don'ts

- If your brows are too thick – do have a professional brow-shaping session in a salon. Once you have the desired shape it is then easier to maintain yourself.

- If your brows are unruly – don't snip off the straggly tops of brows, it does make brows look sharper, but it's easy to make mistakes, so leave it to the professionals.

- When applying your make-up – don't overdo eyebrow colour. Over-defined eyebrows in a colour that is too dark can make you look like a clown. Keep colours soft and suitable for your natural colouring.

now put it all
together.
Here is an easy-to-wear,
basic eye make
for you to
try yourself.

step-by

tep eyes

Prime the eyelids, pick up a little powder on a shadow brush and stroke inwards over the lids. For the most flattering, wide-awake look, the depth of colour should be

darkest at the outer corners, while the inner corners should be almost bare. Blend. Then just with your fingertip add a hint of shimmer to the brow-bone, and blend again.

step 1

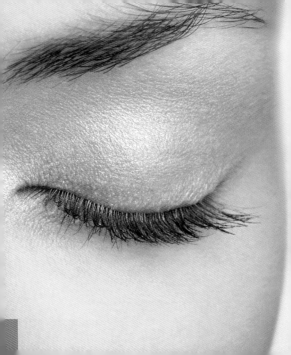

Trace kohl pencil lightly along the lash-line, starting a third of the way from the inner corners on both the upper and lower lids and moving outwards. Use an eye-liner brush or sponge-tipped applicator to smudge and blend the liner well into the lash roots to achieve a softly defined blur.

108

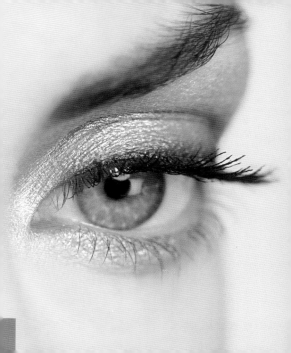

For perfect mascara application, curl your eyelashes first so they are neat, then close the upper lids slowly and firmly onto the mascara wand, forcing the colour consistently through the lashes. Wait for the first coat to dry. Then look up and run the tip of the wand back and forth along the lower lashes. Allow to dry, then brush or comb through to separate lashes and remove any tiny clumps.

step 3

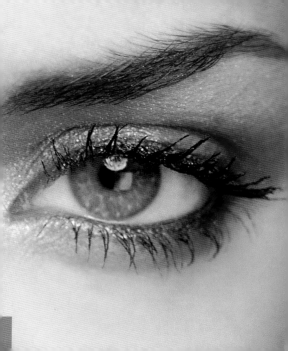

First published in 2000 by
HarperCollins*Illustrated*
An imprint of HarperCollins*Publishers*
77–85 Fulham Palace Road
London W6 8JB

The HarperCollins website address is: www.**fire**and**water**.com

Published in association with The National Magazine Company Limited.
Good Housekeeping is a registered trademark of The National Magazine Company
Limited and the Hearst Corporation.

The Good Housekeeping website is www.goodhousekeeping.co.uk

British Library Cataloguing-in-Publication Data
A catalogue record for this book is available from the British Library.
ISBN 0-00-710444-8
Printed and bound in China by Imago